# the essential bath

Enjoy the benefits
of bathing with essential oils

Penguin Books

Penguin Books Australia Ltd
250 Camberwell Road, Camberwell, Victoria 3124, Australia
Penguin Books Ltd
80 Strand, London WC2R ORL, England
Penguin Putnam Inc.
375 Hudson Street, New York, New York 10014, USA
Penguin Books, a division of Pearson Canada
10 Alcorn Avenue, Toronto, Ontario, Canada M4V 3B2
Penguin Books (NZ) Ltd
Cnr Rosedale and Airborne Roads, Albany, Auckland, New Zealand
Penguin Books (South Africa) (Pty) Ltd
24 Sturdee Avenue, Rosebank, Johannesburg 2196, South Africa
Penguin Books India (P) Ltd
11, Community Centre, Panchsheel Park, New Delhi 110 017, India

First published by Penguin Books Australia Ltd 2003

10 9 8 7 6 5 4 3 2 1

Design by Brad Maxwell, Penguin Design Studio
Cover photography by Julie Anne Renouf
Typeset in 9/14 pt Trade Gothic Light by Post Pre-press Group, Brisbane, Queensland
Printed and bound in Australia by McPherson's Printing Group, Maryborough, Victoria

National Library of Australia
Cataloguing-in-Publication data:

The essential bath.
ISBN 0 14 300168 X.
1. Baths. 2. Essences and essential oils.

613.41

www.penguin.com.au

# contents

# introduction

Taking the time to fill the bath and lay back and relax in it is an all too rare treat in today's busy world. Therefore it makes good sense to enhance the bathing experience by enjoying the benefits of *pure* essential oils. Of all our senses smell is the most powerful. Scents affect our emotional state by interacting with the brain's limbic system. Essential oils engulf you in a cloud of heavenly aromas while at the same time pampering and nourishing your skin. Avoid synthetic fragrant oils as these do not offer therapeutic benefits.

Each essential oil has specific characteristics

and their combination can affect your mind, body and spirit in different ways, so knowing which oils to choose is *essential*. This book provides tips on how to make the most of bathing, useful information about essential oils and simple recipes for you to make depending on your desired result. It also recommends a top ten list of *essential* essential oils (see p 8). If you enjoy the experience then take the time to build your own collection of essential oils, and have fun working your way through the recipes.

# *e*ssentials of bathing

## step by step

To maximise your bathing experience take the phone off the hook, shut the door, light some candles and put on your favourite music. Be sure the bathroom is warm and that you have fresh, soft towels ready for when you step out. Fill the bath before adding your selection of oils. Use a maximum of 10 drops, swish the water around and then slide in. You should allow yourself plenty of time to soak before using soap, as soap will form a barrier on your skin and diminish the therapeutic

effects of the essential oils. The ideal way to make the most of bathing with essential oil is to shower first to get clean, rinse thoroughly, then step into the bath. To gain the maximum benefit, bathe for a period of 15–30 minutes.

## bath temperature

The temperature of the bath is an important consideration. A warm bath is relaxing and suitable for all of the recipes suggested in this book. Avoid hot baths as they can have a weakening effect. If you feel light-headed at any time reduce the temperature of the water or carefully remove yourself from the bath but be sure not to stand up too quickly. Cool baths are invigorating, however, if you do not wish to have a cool bath but feel the need of a lift, take a warm bath, using your essential oils, followed by a quick cool shower. Be sure to re-hydrate whilst bathing by drinking either water or herbal tea.

## shower method

Not everyone has the luxury of a bath in their house, however, it is possible to use the recipes that follow in the shower and still reap the benefits. Simply place a few drops of your chosen blend onto a clean, dry face cloth and, just before stepping out of the shower when you are damp and the room is steamy, briskly rub yourself all over with the infused cloth. Wrap yourself in a towel and take a moment to enjoy the aroma of your selected oils.

## top ten essentials

There is no denying that gathering a collection of essential oils is an expensive process. There are, however, some essential oils that are more *essential* than others. If you make these oils the basis of your collection you will find countless ways to create blends for your particular needs. Listed on the following page are our suggested top ten essential oils.

# top ten essentials

Bergamot

Geranium

Lemon

Grapefruit

Lavender

Clary sage

Palma rosa

Sandalwood

Chamomile

Rose

## recipes and storage

In this book you will find a range of essential oil recipes suitable to use at different times of the day, to create different moods and for a variety of health issues. Each recipe lists the essential oils required followed by the quantity of drops to be blended. To make and use the blends as needed, simply add the specified number of drops of each essential oil to the filled bath before you step in. Alternatively, if you wish to keep a supply of your favourite blend on hand then multiply the quantities equally and make up as much or as little of the blend as you like. Store in a small, airtight, dark glass jar with a dropper and make sure you label it.

## safety

Essential oils should never be used undiluted directly on the skin or taken internally.

*Some* essential oils should not be used during pregnancy and there are others that are unsuitable for children. *All* essential oils should be avoided during the first three months of pregnancy unless approved by a professional practitioner.

See pregnancy essentials on page 12 for a list of essential oils suitable to use after the first trimester. If you are pregnant or wish to use essential oils with children *do not* use the recipes in this book without first seeking the advice of a qualified practitioner.

In addition, if you experience heavy menstrual bleeding *do not* use Juniper.

See glossary for safety information on each type of essential oil.

# pregnancy essentials
## (post first trimester)

∾

Lavender

Tangerine

Mandarin

Grapefruit

Geranium

Chamomile

Rose bulgar

Rose maroc

Jasmine

Ylang ylang

If you are pregnant *do not* use the recipes in this book without first seeking the advice of a qualified practitioner.

# day in,
# day out

This collection of recipes will have you up and out the door in the morning and keep you calm, relaxed and confident throughout the day.

# Wake up call

For a sweet and refreshing start to your morning try
this lively blend of citrus and cardamom.

| | |
|---|---|
| Grapefruit | 3 |
| Lemon | 2 |
| Lime | 1 |
| Cardamom | 1 |

# Smiling start

Step out into the day with a serene smile feeling refreshed and ready for anything.

| | |
|---|---|
| Bergamot | 3 |
| Sandalwood | 2 |
| Basil | 1 |

# Marvellous morn

Wake up your mind with this zesty blend and feel
confident and capable.

| | |
|---|---|
| Grapefruit | 2 |
| Niaouli | 1 |
| Bergamot | 1 |

# Sunbeam

Be transported to one of those glorious blue-sky, gentle breeze kind of days.

| | |
|---|---|
| Petigrain | 2 |
| Camphor | 1 |
| Palma rosa | 1 |

# Cloak of clarity

If your day is full of meetings or public speaking, shroud yourself in a mantle of confidence and be heard.

| | |
|---|---|
| Palma rosa | 3 |
| Bergamot | 2 |
| Clary sage | 1 |

# Courage

These warm, soothing and spicy oils will ensure you feel undaunted when facing a new situation or meeting new people.

| | |
|---|---|
| Ginger | 3 |
| Black pepper | 1 |
| Clove | 1 |

# Aromatic alignment

If you are finding it difficult to make a decision or to focus, this blend will gently redirect your mind.

| | |
|---|---|
| Orange | 3 |
| Niaouli | 2 |
| Cardamom | 1 |

# party mood

When you have plans for the evening after a busy day, here is a selection of recipes to put the zing back into your step and leave you feeling like the life of the party.

# Spirit of revival

Revive your spirits after an exhausting day.

| | |
|---|---|
| Lemon | 4 |
| Bergamot | 2 |
| Rosemary | 1 |

# Counterbalance

The pressures of the day will disappear from your mind.

| | |
|---|---|
| Ginger | 2 |
| Lavender | 1 |

# Renewal

Spend some time in a forest before stepping back into the world.

| | |
|---|---|
| Sandalwood | 3 |
| Eucalyptus | 2 |

# Top gear

Banish lethargy and fast-track your way to a night of fun.

| | |
|---|---|
| Clary sage | 3 |
| Bergamot | 3 |
| Geranium | 1 |

## Party flavour

This blend will turn your mood to laughter, dancing
and chatter.

|        |   |
|--------|---|
| Rose   | 4 |
| Lemon  | 3 |
| Ginger | 1 |

# sweet dreams

At the end of a long day pamper yourself with one of these recipes to make the gentle transition from activity to relaxation.

# Safe haven

When you are finally home to stay, allow yourself to
be carried to bed by this blend.

| | |
|---|---|
| Petigrain | 3 |
| Clary sage | 2 |

# Floral consolation

These healing aromas clear your mind and encourage a sleep free of worry.

| | |
|---|---|
| Geranium | 2 |
| Lemon | 2 |
| Ylang ylang | 1 |
| Rose | 1 |

# Mermaid's bath

Imagine you are a glorious sea-creature and feel the stresses and pressures float away.

| | |
|---|---|
| Clary sage | 2 |
| Orange | 2 |
| Marjoram | 1 |

# Sanctuary

Escape from the hectic pace of daily life into this relaxing blend.

| | |
|---|---|
| Sandalwood | 2 |
| Rose | 2 |
| Petigrain | 1 |

# Serene slumber

Sleep peacefully and allow your body and mind to regenerate.

| | |
|---|---|
| Rose maroc | 2 |
| Jasmine | 1 |
| Chamomile | 1 |

# Sweet dreams

Transport yourself through your imagination to a secret hideaway.

| | |
|---|---|
| Sandalwood | 3 |
| Lemon | 1 |
| Chamomile | 1 |

# Peace

Centre yourself while you soak in this blend and enjoy a peaceful sleep.

| Neroli | 3 |
| Rose | 2 |
| Lime | 1 |
| Ylang ylang | 1 |

# stress busters

A bath can be a sanctuary from the demands of modern living. With the addition of specially chosen essential oils, this relaxing ritual can ease stress and tension and re-centre your mind.

# First aid

When you are at the end of your endurance shut the door on the world and slide into this bath.

| | |
|---|---|
| Sandalwood | 3 |
| Geranium | 2 |
| Lavender | 1 |

# Pressure valve

Feel the pressures flowing out from your body through your fingertips and toes.

| | |
|---|---|
| Bergamot | 3 |
| Grapefruit | 1 |
| Basil | 1 |

# Anxiety ease

Imagine the scents you breathe calming your mind.

| | |
|---|---|
| Lavender | 2 |
| Geranium | 2 |
| Palma rosa | 2 |

# Emotional balm

When it all gets too much, wrap yourself up in this
soothing blend.

| | |
|---|---|
| Sandalwood | 3 |
| Rose maroc | 1 |
| Cardamom | 1 |

# Watery retreat

Retreat into a soothing bath and feel the worries of the world drain away.

| | |
|---|---|
| Chamomile | 4 |
| Bergamot | 2 |

## Liquid fortitude

When you wake up feeling overwhelmed by all that is ahead of you, take time to prepare for the day.

| | |
|---|---|
| Rose | 3 |
| Grapefruit | 3 |
| Neroli | 1 |

# Appetite

Loss of appetite due to emotional stress is common.
Give your digestive system a gentle hand by bathing
in this warmly scented blend.

| | |
|---|---|
| Neroli | 2 |
| Chamomile | 2 |

# healing

These specially blended recipes are based on the
ancient tradition of healing baths, however they
should not be seen as an alternative to seeking the
opinion of a trained health practitioner.

# Headache

Relax in this soothing blend and feel the pressure ease.

| | |
|---|---|
| Lavender | 3 |
| Chamomile | 1 |

# Sinus pain

Wrap yourself in this aroma to release the pressure in your head.

| | |
|---|---|
| Rosemary | 2 |
| Geranium | 1 |
| Eucalyptus | 1 |

# Head cold

Relieve the congestion with this healthy blend and breathe more easily.

| | |
|---|---|
| Lemon | 2 |
| Tea-tree | 2 |
| Cinnamon | 1 |
| Eucalyptus | 1 |

# Flu

This blend will ease the aches and pains.

| | |
|---|---|
| Tea-tree | 3 |
| Lavender | 2 |
| Thyme | 1 |
| Cinnamon | 1 |

# Muscular aches

Bathe in this delicious blend and feel your aches disappear.

| Lemon | 2 |
| Clary sage | 2 |
| Orange | 1 |

## Post workout

Take this bath before going to bed to ease muscular
pain and ensure a good night's sleep.

| Lavender | 4 |
| Ginger | 3 |

# Detox

This will leave you feeling as though you have jumped into a bath of tiny toxin eradicators. For added benefit, drink a glass of water before and after you bathe.

| | |
|---|---|
| Grapefruit | 3 |
| Lemon | 2 |
| Lime | 1 |
| Rosemary | 1 |

# Hangover

Bathe with this blend and treat yourself to a quiet day of recovery.

| | |
|---|---|
| Lemon | 3 |
| Fennel | 2 |
| Sandalwood | 2 |
| Lavender | 1 |

# Hangover terror

It's the morning after a big night and you need to be fresh to face the day ahead.

| | |
|---|---|
| Grapefruit | 3 |
| Fennel | 2 |
| Rosemary | 1 |
| Lemon | 1 |

# Chills

When you just can't get warm, hop into this bath and have warm towels and snuggly socks at the ready.

| Ginger | 3 |
| Geranium | 2 |

# Sun-splashed

Replenish and soothe your skin after a day in the sun by massaging your body as you relax in this bath.

| | |
|---|---|
| Chamomile | 4 |
| Geranium | 2 |
| Lavender | 2 |

# hormonal
# harmony

Changing hormone levels affect women differently. If you experience premenstrual symptoms, take time to relax with these essential oils and feel more in balance.

# Short fuse

Nurture yourself in this soothing blend and count to ten.

| | |
|---|---|
| Palma rosa | 3 |
| Bergamot | 3 |
| Geranium | 3 |

# Handle with care

Balance your changing moods with this uplifting
bath.

| | |
|---|---|
| Clary sage | 3 |
| Geranium | 1 |
| Bergamot | 1 |

# Cranky pants

Hang 'do not disturb' on the door and retire to your sanctuary.

| | |
|---|---|
| Bergamot | 3 |
| Chamomile | 2 |
| Geranium | 1 |

# Low energy

Take the time to treat yourself to this refreshing blend of oils.

| Grapefruit | 3 |
| Clary sage | 2 |

# Period pain

Wrap yourself in this cocoon of scents and feel the
discomfort ease away.

| | |
|---|---|
| Palma rosa | 3 |
| Neroli | 2 |
| Clary sage | 2 |

# pure indulgence

Treat your body and mind with care and attention and you will reap the benefits – so lie back and enjoy these indulgent recipes.

# Serene princess

Serenity will radiate from within as you centre your soul and mind with this blend.

| | |
|---|---|
| Petigrain | 2 |
| Rosewood | 2 |
| Tangerine | 2 |

# Sweet serenade

This heady mix will gently enfold you in its sweet bouquet.

| | |
|---|---|
| Orange | 3 |
| Lavender | 3 |
| Geranium | 2 |

# Body toner

The astringent quality of this blend will stimulate, detoxify and tone your skin.

| Grapefruit | 3 |
| Neroli | 2 |
| Juniper | 2 |

# Goddess

When *you* believe you're special, so will others.

| | |
|---|---|
| Ylang ylang | 3 |
| Geranium | 2 |
| Cardamom | 1 |
| Chamomile | 1 |

# Indulgence

Treat your body to this cleansing blend and transform bathing into a celebration of pleasure.

| | |
|---|---|
| Neroli | 2 |
| Sandalwood | 2 |
| Rose | 1 |

# passion palace

Create a special atmosphere with candles, music and champagne when you are planning a bath with your lover. Then choose one of these recipes to start the sparks flying.

# Love potion

Nurture yourself with this blend and draw love from those around you.

| | |
|---|---|
| Palma rosa | 4 |
| Ylang ylang | 1 |
| Ginger | 1 |
| Rosemary | 1 |
| Cardamom | 1 |

# Sexual energy

Have fun, go wild, play new games with your beloved.

| | |
|---|---|
| Ginger | 2 |
| Patchouli | 2 |
| Cardamom | 1 |
| Sandalwood | 1 |

# Seduction

You are a woman on a mission – bathe in this rich, complex blend and know that you are irresistible.

| | |
|---|---|
| Jasmine | 3 |
| Rose | 2 |
| Mandarin | 1 |

# Passion

Ignite the senses and surrender to the mood.

| | |
|---|---|
| Rose | 3 |
| Palma rosa | 2 |
| Nutmeg | 1 |

# Heady

This rich, complex scent is pure passion – allow it to flood your senses.

| | |
|---|---|
| Sandalwood | 3 |
| Patchouli | 2 |
| Rose | 1 |

# glossary

# Basil

*(Ocimum basilicum)*

The peppery scented basil oil has therapeutic applications for colds, fatigue, lack of concentration and headaches.

Safety: Avoid during pregnancy; can irritate sensitive skins.

# Bergamot

*(Citrus bergamia)*

Bergamot is effective for conditions such as stress, anxiety, mood swings, worry and depression. This oil uplifts and soothes.

Safety: Phototoxic, do not expose the skin to sun for twelve hours after use.

# Black pepper

*(Piper nigrum)*

An excellent remedy for chills and poor circulation, as well as muscular aches. It is believed to have aphrodisiac qualities and has been used to treat sexual disharmony and impotence.

Safety: Non-toxic, non-irritant.

# Camphor

*(Cinnamomum camphora)*

Camphor is effective in the relief of symptoms of colds, coughs, fever and aches.
Safety: Non-toxic, non-irritant.

# Cardamom

*(Elettaria cardamomum)*

Cardamom helps to alleviate digestive, circulatory and respiratory complaints. It can also assist in stimulating the appetite.

Safety: Non-toxic, non-irritant, non-sensitising.

## Chamomile

*(Anthemis nobilis)*

Extremely soothing and gentle, chamomile is suitable for use with children. Effective in the relief of sunburn, rashes and allergies as well as headaches, migraine and stress.

Safety: Non-toxic, non-irritant.

# Cinnamon

*(Cinnamomum zeylanicum)*

Cinnamon is useful in fighting colds, viral infection, congestion or flu.

Safety: Leaf oil is considered to be non-toxic. Bark oil should be used with caution as it is stronger and not recommended for skin care.

## Clary sage

*(Salvia sclarea)*

Clary sage is particularly beneficial for women due to its antispasmodic effect which lowers blood pressure, relieves menstrual migraine, eases PMS and rejuvenates the skin. The aroma of clary sage is also very uplifting.

Safety: Non-toxic. Do not use during pregnancy.

# Clove

*(Eugenis caryphllus)*

Clove has a mildly anaesthetic effect; it can be used to stimulate digestion and restore appetite. It also aids concentration.

Safety: Use in small quantities as it can cause skin irritation.

# Eucalyptus

*(Eucalyptus globulus)*

Effective in treating the symptoms of colds and flu,
eucalyptus also relieves muscular aches and assists
with skin infections.
Safety: Non-toxic, non-irritant.

# Fennel

*(Foeniculum vulgare)*

Fennel's spicy fresh aroma improves concentration and eases lethargy and muscular aches.

Safety: Non-toxic, non-irritant.

## Geranium

*(Pelargonium graveolens)*

Geranium is an excellent balm for combination and mature skins. It acts as an antidepressant and can ease premenstrual tension.

Safety: Non-toxic, non-irritant.

# Ginger

*(Zingiber officinale)*

Ginger aids digestion, blood circulation and combats bloating. It has a beneficial effect on energy and confidence.

Safety: Non-toxic, non-irritant.

# Grapefruit

*(Citrus paradisi)*

Grapefruit is a stimulating and uplifting oil and is effective against nervous exhaustion and depression. It also stimulates the lymphatic system. Safety: Non-toxic, non-irritant, non-sensitising.

# Jasmine

*(Jasminum officinale)*

Jasmine rejuvenates skin and is considered an aphrodisiac. It acts as an antispasmodic, and can be used during labour and also to stimulate breast milk.

Safety: Non-toxic. Do not use during pregnancy.

# Juniper

*(Juniperus communis)*

Juniper combats muscular aches and pains and can also act to relieve mental fatigue and anxiety. Safety: Non-toxic. Do not use during pregnancy or if you are subject to heavy menstrual bleeding.

# Lavender

*(Lavandula angustifolia)*

Lavender is effective as an antiseptic and can be used to treat bites, cuts and burns. It has pain-killing properties and eases muscular aches, headaches and migraine.

Safety: Non-toxic, non-irritant.

# Lemon

*(Citrus limonum)*

A great detoxifier, lemon's fresh aroma revives and lifts your mood. It can ease congestion and relieve the symptoms of colds and flu.

Safety: Phototoxic, do not expose the skin to sunlight for twelve hours after use.

# Lime

*(Citrus aurantifolia)*

The refreshing scent of lime makes it a useful antidote to feelings of depression, stress, anxiety and apathy. This antiseptic oil can also work to stimulate digestion.

Safety: Non-toxic, non-irritant, non-sensitising. Cold-pressed oil is phototoxic.

# Mandarin

*(Citris nobilis)*

This antiseptic oil is beneficial for the skin, particularly in the treatment of acne and scars. Mandarin's sweet, fruity aroma refreshes and soothes the mind and body.

Safety: Non-toxic, non-sensitising.

# Marjoram

## (Origanum majorana)

Marjoram relieves muscular aches and pains and is useful for combating anxiety and insomnia.

Safety: Non-toxic, non-irritant.

# Niaouli

*(Melaleuca quinquenervia)*

Niaouli has antiseptic qualities. It is effective in treating cuts and infections as well as acne.
Safety: Non-toxic, non-irritant, non-sensitising.

# Neroli

### *(Citrus aurantium, amara)*

Derived from orange blossom, neroli is an effective antidote to panic and shock. It is also useful in healing scar tissue. Particularly suited to sensitive skin types.

Safety: Non-toxic, non-irritant.

# Orange

*(Citrus sinensis)*

A gentle stress reliever, orange also improves digestion and is a great tonic for acne.
Safety: Non-toxic, non-irritant.

## Palma rosa

*(Cymbopogon martinii)*

This sweet, slightly lemon-scented oil is antifungal and soothes dry or inflamed skin. It is also useful for treating depression, insomnia and nervous exhaustion.

Safety: Non-toxic, non-irritant.

## Patchouli

*(Pogostemon cablin)*

Patchouli has an earthy rich scent that helps to calm and ground an exhausted mind. It is also an excellent skin tonic, relieving dry, chapped skin, and is considered an aphrodisiac.

Safety: Non-toxic, non-irritant.

# Petigrain

*(Citrus aurantium)*

Petigrain can be useful against exhaustion, insomnia and stress as it works to calm and restore balance and mental clarity.

Safety: Non-toxic, non-irritant, non-sensitising.

# Rose

*(Rosa damascena)*

Rose has antispasmodic properties and works as a liver tonic and skin rejuvenator. It eases mental tension, insomnia and lessens feelings of grief, anger or helplessness.

Safety: Non-toxic, non-irritant.

# Rosemary

*(Rosmarinus officinalis)*

Rosemary oil improves concentration, relieves muscular aches and pains and reduces fluid retention.

Safety: Generally non-toxic, non-irritant. Not advised for epileptics.

# Sandalwood

*(Santalum album)*

Sandalwood has been treasured for thousands of years for its spicy aroma which is intensely relaxing and calming.

Safety: Non-toxic, non-irritant.

# Tea-tree

*(Melaleuca alternifolia)*

Tea-tree is antifungal, antibacterial, antiseptic and antiviral, and is effective in relieving the symptoms of colds and flu.

Safety: Non-toxic, non-irritant.

# Ylang ylang

*(Cananga odorata)*

Ylang ylang is effective for nervous tension, anxiety and mood swings. This deeply relaxing oil is thought to be an aphrodisiac, however its heady floral scent can cause headaches.

Safety: Non-toxic.

# the essential bath